The Ultimate Mediterranean Dash Diet Recipe Collection

Don't Miss These Quick and Easy Recipes to Make Incredible Mediterranean Dash Diet Meals

Kathyrn Solano

© Copyright 2021 - All rights reserved.

The content contained within this book may not be reproduced, duplicated or transmitted without direct written permission from the author or the publisher.

Under no circumstances will any blame or legal responsibility be held against the publisher, or author, for any damages, reparation, or monetary loss due to the information contained within this book. Either directly or indirectly.

Legal Notice:

This book is copyright protected. This book is only for personal use. You cannot amend, distribute, sell, use, quote or paraphrase any part, or the content within this book, without the consent of the author or publisher.

Disclaimer Notice:

Please note the information contained within this document is for educational and entertainment purposes only. All effort has been executed to present accurate, up to date, and reliable, complete information. No warranties of any kind are declared or implied. Readers acknowledge that the author is not engaging in the rendering of legal, financial, medical or professional advice. The content within this book has been derived from various sources. Please consult a licensed professional before attempting any techniques outlined in this book.

By reading this document, the reader agrees that under no circumstances is the author responsible for any losses, direct or indirect, which are incurred as a result of the use of information contained within this document, including, but not limited to, — errors, omissions, or inaccuracies.

Table of contents

LUNCH AND DINNER RECIPES 6

- BEAN LETTUCE WRAPS 6
- GREEK CHICKEN SHISH KEBAB 8
- SKILLET SHRIMP WITH SUMMER SQUASH AND CHORIZO 10
- SHRIMP & PENNE 13
- CHICKPEAS AND BRUSSEL SPROUTS SALAD 15
- MEAT LOAF 16
- COUSCOUS WITH PEPPERONCINI & TUNA 18
- TILAPIA WITH AVOCADO & RED ONION 20
- BAKED SALMON WITH DILL 22
- DELICIOUS BROCCOLI TORTELLINI SALAD 23
- MIXED SPICE BURGERS 25
- CRISPY BAKED CHICKEN 27
- MILANO CHICKEN 29
- ITALIAN BAKED BEANS 31
- TOMATO TILAPIA 33
- BACON WRAPPED ASPARAGUS 35
- MOROCCAN SPICED STIR-FRIED BEEF WITH BUTTERNUT SQUASH AND CHICKPEAS 37
- HERB-CRUSTED HALIBUT 40
- SYRIAN SPICED LENTIL, BARLEY, AND VEGETABLE SOUP 42
- SPINACH CHICKEN 44
- NIÇOISE-STYLE TUNA SALAD WITH OLIVES & WHITE BEANS 46
- WHOLE-WHEAT PASTA WITH ROASTED RED PEPPER SAUCE AND FRESH MOZZARELLA 48
- GREEK TURKEY MEATBALL GYRO WITH TZATZIKI 50
- GRILLED MEDITERRANEAN CHICKEN KEBABS 53
- KIDNEY BEANS CILANTRO SALAD 56
- BARLEY AND MUSHROOM SOUP 58
- PAN-SEARED SCALLOPS WITH PEPPER & ONIONS IN ANCHOVY OIL ... 60
- SPINACH SALAD WITH BLOOD ORANGE VINAIGRETTE 62
- LASAGNA TORTELLINI SOUP 65
- GREEK QUINOA BOWLS 68
- SALMON STEW 71
- BALSAMIC CHICKEN AND VEGGIE SKEWERS 73
- PESTO CHICKEN AND TOMATO ZOODLES 76

Broiled Herb Sole With Cauliflower Mashed Potatoes 78
   Citrus Poached Lovely Salmon 81

GREAT MEDITERRANEAN DIET RECIPES 83
   Herb rice 83
   Pecorino pasta with sausage and tomato 85
   Pesto pasta and shrimp 87
   Feta tomato sea bass 89
   Bulgur Vegetable Salad 91
   Cauliflower Breadsticks 92
   Cheesecake Ice Cream 93
   Vanilla Custard 94
   Chocolate Fruit Kebabs 95

SAUCES AND DRESSINGS RECIPES 97
   Chunky Roasted Cherry Tomato And Basil Sauce 97
   Basil, Almond, And Celery Heart Pesto 99
   Sweet And Spicy Green Pumpkin Seeds 101
   Chermoula Sauce 103
   Pesto Deviled Eggs With Sun-dried Tomatoes 105
   North African Spiced Sautéed Cabbage 107

LUNCH AND DINNER RECIPES

Bean Lettuce Wraps

Servings: 4

Cooking Time: 20 Minutes

Ingredients:

8 Romaine lettuce leaves

½ cup Garlic hummus or any prepared hummus

¾ cup chopped tomatoes

15 ounce can great northern beans, drained and rinsed

½ cup diced onion

1 tablespoon extra virgin olive oil

¼ cup chopped parsley

¼ teaspoon black pepper

Directions:

Set a skillet on top of the stove range over medium heat.

In the skillet, warm the oil for a couple of minutes.

Add the onion into the oil. Stir frequently as the onion cooks for a few minutes.

Combine the pepper and tomatoes and cook for another couple of minutes. Remember to stir occasionally.

Add the beans and continue to stir and cook for 2 to 3 minutes.

Turn the burner off, remove the skillet from heat, and add the parsley.

Set the lettuce leaves on a flat surface and spread 1 tablespoon of hummus on each leaf.

Divide the bean mixture onto the leaves.

Spread the bean mixture down the center of the leaves.

Fold the leaves by starting lengthwise on one side.

Fold over the other side so the leaf is completely wrapped.

Serve and enjoy!

Nutrition Info: calories: 211, fats: 8 grams, carbohydrates: 28 grams, protein: 10 grams.

Greek Chicken Shish Kebab

Servings: 6

Cooking Time: 10 Minutes

Ingredients:

¼ cup olive oil

¼ cup lemon juice

¼ cup white vinegar

2 garlic cloves, minced

1 teaspoon ground cumin

1 teaspoon dried oregano

½ teaspoon dried thyme

¼ teaspoon salt

¼ teaspoon ground black pepper

2 pounds boneless and skinless chicken breasts, cut up into 1½inch pieces

6 wooden skewers

2 large green or red bell peppers, cut up into 1inch pieces

12 cherry tomatoes

12 fresh mushrooms

Directions:

In a large bowl, whisk in olive oil, vinegar, garlic, lemon juice, cumin, thyme, oregano, salt, and black pepper. Mix well. Add the chicken to the bowl and coat it thoroughly by tossing it. Cover the bowl with plastic wrap, refrigerate, and allow it to marinate for 2 hours.

Soak your wooden skewers in water for about 30 minutes. Preheat grill to medium-high heat and lightly oil the grate. Remove the chicken from your marinade and shake off any extra liquid. Discard the remaining marinade. Thread pieces of chicken with bits of onion, bell pepper, cherry tomatoes, and mushrooms alternating between them. Cook on grill for 10 minutes each side until browned on all sides. Chill, place to containers. Pre-heat before eating. Enjoy!

Nutrition Info: Calories: 183, Total Fat: 9.8 g, Saturated Fat: 1.4 g, Cholesterol: 22 mg, Sodium: 141 mg, Total Carbohydrate: 14.1 g, Dietary Fiber: 4.4 g, Total Sugars: 8.5 g, Protein: 6 g, Vitamin D: 130 mcg, Calcium: 42 mg, Iron: 3 mg, Potassium: 821 mg

Skillet Shrimp With Summer Squash And Chorizo

Servings: 8
Cooking Time: 20 Minutes

Ingredients:

1 lb large shrimp or prawns, peeled and deveined, tail can remain or frozen frozen, thawed

7 oz Spanish Chorizo, or mild Chorizo or hot Chorizo, sliced

Extra virgin olive oil

Juice of 1/2 lemon

1 summer squash, halved then sliced, half moons

1 small hot pepper such as jalapeno pepper, optional

1/2 medium red onion, sliced

Fresh parsley for garnish

3/4 tsp smoked paprika

3/4 tsp ground cumin

1/2 tsp garlic powder

Salt, to taste

Pepper, to taste

Directions:

Pat shrimp dry, then season with salt, pepper, paprika, cumin, and garlic powder, toss to coat, set aside

In a large cast iron skillet over medium-high, add the Chorizo and brown on both sides, about 4 minutes or until the Chorizo is cooked, transfer to a plate

In the same skillet, add a drizzle of extra virgin olive oil if needed

Add the summer squash, and a sprinkle of salt and pepper and sear undisturbed for about 3 to minutes on one side. turnover and sear another 2 minutes on the other side until nicely colored, transfer the squash to the plate with Chorizo

In the same skillet, now add a little extra virgin olive oil and tilting to make sure the bottom is well coated

Once heated, add the shrimp and cook, stirring frequently, until the shrimp flesh starts to turn a little pink, but still not quite fully cooked, about 3 minutes

Return the Chorizo and squash to the skillet, toss to combine, cook another 3 minutes or until shrimp is cooked – its pink and the tails turn a bright red

Transfer the shrimp skillet to a large serving platter, allow to cool

Distribute among the containers, store for 2-3 days

To Serve: Reheat on the stove for 1-2 minutes or until heated through. Squeeze 1/2 lemon on top, and sliced red onions and hot peppers.

Nutrition Info: Calories:192;Carbs: 4g;Total Fat:; Protein: 17g

Shrimp & Penne

Servings: 8

Cooking Time: 35 Minutes

Ingredients:

Penne pasta (16 oz. pkg.)

Salt (.25 tsp.)

Olive oil (2 tbsp.)

Diced tomatoes (2 - 14.5 oz. cans)

Garlic (1 tbsp.)

Red onion (.25 cup)

White wine (.25 cup)

Shrimp (1 lb.)

Grated parmesan cheese (1 cup)

Directions:

Dice the red onion and garlic. Peel and devein the shrimp.

Add salt to a large soup pot of water and set it on the stovetop to boil. Add the pasta and cook for nine to ten minutes. Drain it thoroughly in a colander.

Empty oil into a skillet. Warm it using the medium temperature setting.

Toss in the garlic and onion to sauté until they're tender.

Pour in the tomatoes and wine. Continue cooking for about ten minutes, stirring occasionally.

Fold in the shrimp and continue cooking for about five minutes or until it's opaque.

Combine the pasta and shrimp and top it off with the cheese to serve.

Nutrition Info: Calories: 3 ;Fat: 8.5 grams; Protein: 24.5 grams

Chickpeas And Brussel Sprouts Salad

Servings: 4

Cooking Time: 10 Minutes

Ingredients:

1 cup roasted chickpeas. To give the dish a saltier taste, you can add sea salt.

4 cups kale, chopped

9 ounces Brussels sprouts, shredded

1 avocado, peeled, pitted, and cut

Directions:

Divide the kale and Brussels sprouts into four bowls.

Add the chickpeas and the avocado.

You can add a little sea salt and/or pepper to taste. Another tip for more taste is to drizzle a little Vinaigrette dressing or your favorite homemade Mediterranean dressing.

Nutrition Info: calories: 337, fats: 20 grams, carbohydrates: 30 grams, protein: 12 grams.

Meat Loaf

Servings: 12

Cooking Time: 1 Hour 15 Minutes

Ingredients:

1 garlic clove, minced

½ teaspoon dried thyme, crushed

½ pound grass-fed lean ground beef

1 organic egg, beaten

Salt and black pepper, to taste

¼ cup onions, chopped

1/8 cup sugar-free ketchup

2 cups mozzarella cheese, freshly grated

¼ cup green bell pepper, seeded and chopped

½ cup cheddar cheese, grated

1 cup fresh spinach, chopped

Directions:

Preheat the oven to 350 degrees F and grease a baking dish.

Put all the ingredients in a bowl except spinach and cheese and mix well.

Arrange the meat over a wax paper and top with spinach and cheese.

Roll the paper around the mixture to form a meatloaf.

Remove the wax paper and transfer the meat loaf in the baking dish.

Put it in the oven and bake for about 1 hour.

Dish out and serve hot.

Meal Prep Tip: Let the meat loafs cool for about 10 minutes to bring them to room temperature before serving.

Nutrition Info: Calories: 43;Carbohydrates: 8g;Protein: 40.8g;Fat: 26g ;Sugar: 1.6g;Sodium: 587mg

Couscous With Pepperoncini & Tuna

Servings: 4

Cooking Time: 20 Minutes

Ingredients:

The Couscous:

Chicken broth or water (1 cup)

Couscous (1.25 cups)

Kosher salt (.75 tsp.)

The Accompaniments:

Oil-packed tuna (2- 5-oz. cans)

Cherry tomatoes (1 pint - halved)

Sliced pepperoncini (.5 cup)

Chopped fresh parsley (.33 cup)

Capers (.25 cup)

Olive oil (for serving)

Black pepper & kosher salt (as desired)

Lemon (1 quartered)

Directions:

Make the couscous in a small saucepan using water or broth. Prepare it using the medium heat temperature setting. Let it sit for about ten minutes.

Toss the tomatoes, tuna, capers, parsley, and pepperoncini into a mixing bowl.

Fluff the couscous when done and dust using the pepper and salt. Spritz it using the oil and serve with the tuna mix and a lemon wedge.

Nutrition Info: Calories: 226;Protein: 8 grams; Fat: 1 gram

Tilapia With Avocado & Red Onion

Servings: 4

Cooking Time: 15 Minutes

Ingredients:

Olive oil (1 tbsp.)

Sea salt (.25 tsp.)

Fresh orange juice (1 tbsp.)

Tilapia fillets (four 4 oz. - more rectangular than square)

Red onion (.25 cup)

Sliced avocado (1)

Also Needed: 9-inch pie plate

Directions:

Combine the salt, juice, and oil to add into the pie dish. Work with one fillet at a time. Place it in the dish and turn to coat all sides.

Arrange the fillets in a wagon wheel-shaped formation. (Each of the fillets should be in the center of the dish with the other end draped over the edge.

Place a tablespoon of the onion on top of each of the fillets and fold the end into the center. Cover the dish with plastic wrap, leaving one corner open to vent the steam.

Place in the microwave using the high heat setting for three minutes. It's done when the center can be easily flaked.

Top the fillets off with avocado and serve.

Nutrition Info: Calories: 200;Protein: 22 grams; Fat: 11 grams

Baked Salmon With Dill

Servings: 4

Cooking Time: 15 Minutes

Ingredients:

Salmon fillets (4- 6 oz. portions - 1-inch thickness)

Kosher salt (.5 tsp.)

Finely chopped fresh dill (1.5 tbsp.)

Black pepper (.125 tsp.)

Lemon wedges (4)

Directions:

Warm the oven in advance to reach 350° Fahrenheit. Lightly grease a baking sheet with a misting of cooking oil spray and add the fish. Lightly spritz the fish with the spray along with a shake of salt, pepper, and dill.

Bake it until the fish is easily flaked (10 min..)

Serve with lemon wedges.

Nutrition Info: Calories: 2;Protein: 28 grams; Fat: 16 grams

Delicious Broccoli Tortellini Salad

Servings: 12

Cooking Time: 20 To 25 Minutes

Ingredients:

1 cup sunflower seeds, or any of your favorite seeds

3 heads of broccoli, fresh is best!

½ cup sugar

20 ounces cheese-filled tortellini

1 onion

2 teaspoons cider vinegar

½ cup mayonnaise

1 cup raisins-optional

Directions:

Cut your broccoli into florets and chop the onion.

Follow the directions to make the cheese-filled tortellini. Once they are cooked, drain and rinse them with cold water.

In a bowl, combine your mayonnaise, sugar, and vinegar. Whisk well to give the ingredients a dressing consistency.

In a separate large bowl, toss in your seeds, onion, tortellini, raisins, and broccoli.

Pour the salad dressing into the large bowl and toss the ingredients together. You will want to ensure everything is thoroughly mixed as you'll want a taste of the salad dressing with every bite!

Nutrition Info: calories: 272, fats: 8.1 grams, carbohydrates: 38. grams, protein: 5 grams.

Mixed Spice Burgers

Servings: 6/2 Chops Each

Cooking Time: 25-30 Minutes

Ingredients:

Medium onion (1)

Fresh parsley (3 tbsp.)

Clove of garlic (1)

Ground allspice (.75 tsp.)

Pepper (.75 tsp.)

Ground nutmeg (.25 tsp.)

Cinnamon (.5 tsp.)

Salt (.5 tsp.)

Fresh mint (2 tbsp.)

90% lean ground beef (1.5 lb.)

Optional: Cold Tzatziki sauce

Directions:

Finely chop/mince the parsley, mint, garlic, and onions. Whisk the nutmeg, salt, cinnamon, pepper, allspice, garlic, mint, parsley, and onion.

Add the beef and prepare six (6 2x4-inch oblong patties.

Use the medium temperature setting to grill the patties or broil them four inches from the heat source for four to six minutes per side.

When they're done, the meat thermometer will register 160° Fahrenheit. Serve with the sauce if desired.

Nutrition Info: Calories: 231; Protein: 32 grams; Fat: 9 grams

Crispy Baked Chicken

Servings: 2

Cooking Time: 40 Minutes

Ingredients:

2 chicken breasts, skinless and boneless

2 tablespoons butter

¼ teaspoon turmeric powder

Salt and black pepper, to taste

¼ cup sour cream

Directions:

Preheat the oven to 360 degrees F and grease a baking dish with butter.

Season the chicken with turmeric powder, salt and black pepper in a bowl.

Put the chicken on the baking dish and transfer it in the oven.

Bake for about 10 minutes and dish out to serve topped with sour cream.

Transfer the chicken in a bowl and set aside to cool for meal prepping.

Divide it into 2 containers and cover the containers. Refrigerate for up to 2 days and reheat in microwave before serving.

Nutrition Info: Calories: 304 ;Carbohydrates: 1.4g;Protein: 21g;Fat: 21.6g ;Sugar: 0.1g;Sodium: 137mg

Milano Chicken

Servings: 6

Cooking Time: 30 Minutes

Ingredients:

4 skinless and boneless chicken breast halves

1 tablespoon vegetable oil

2 garlic cloves, crushed

1 teaspoon Italian style seasoning

1 teaspoon crushed red pepper flakes

salt

pepper

1 28-ounce can stewed drained tomatoes

1 9-ounce package frozen green beans

Directions:

Heat oil in a large skillet over medium-high heat.

Add chicken to the skillet and season with garlic, red pepper, Italian seasoning, salt, and pepper.

Saute for about 5 minutes.

Add tomatoes and cook for 5 minutes more.

Add green beans and give the whole mixture a gentle stir.

Reduce heat, cover, and simmer for about 15-20 minutes.

Enjoy!

Nutrition Info: Calories: 244, Total Fat: 4.9 g, Saturated Fat: 0.5 g, Cholesterol: mg, Sodium: 399 mg, Total Carbohydrate: 14.1 g, Dietary Fiber: 4.6 g, Total Sugars: 6.4 g, Protein: 38.2 g, Vitamin D: 0 mcg, Calcium: 48 mg, Iron: 3 mg, Potassium: 662 mg

Italian Baked Beans

Servings: 6

Cooking Time: 15 To 20 Minutes.

Ingredients:

½ cup chopped onion

¼ cup red wine vinegar

¼ tablespoon ground cinnamon

15 ounces or 2 cans of great northern beans, do not drain

2 teaspoons extra virgin olive oil

12 ounces tomato paste, low sodium

½ cup water

Directions:

Turn a burner to medium heat and add oil to a saucepan.

Add the onion and cook for 4 to 5 minutes. Stir well.

Combine the vinegar, tomato paste, cinnamon, and water. Mix until all the ingredients are well combined. Switch the heat to a low setting.

Using a colander, drain one can of beans and pour into the pan.

Open the second can of beans and pour all of it, including the liquid, into the saucepan and stir.

Continue to cook the beans for 10 minutes while stirring frequently.

Serve and enjoy!

Nutrition Info: calories: 236, fats: 3 grams, carbohydrates: 42 grams, protein: 10 grams.

Tomato Tilapia

Servings: 4

Cooking Time: 15 Minutes

Ingredients:

3 tablespoons sun-dried tomatoes packed in oil, drained (juice/oil reserved) and chopped

1 tablespoon capers, drained

2 pieces tilapia

1 tablespoon oil from sun-dried tomatoes

1 tablespoon lemon juice

2 tablespoons Kalamata olives, pitted and chopped

Directions:

Preheat oven to 375 degrees F.

Add sun-dried tomatoes, capers, and olives to a bowl; stir well and set aside.

Place the tilapia fillets side by side on a baking sheet.

Drizzle with oil and lemon juice.

Bake for about 10-1minutes.

Check the fish after 10 minutes to see if they are flakey.

Once done, top the fish with tomato mixture.

Nutrition Info: Calories: , Total Fat: 4.4 g, Saturated Fat: 0.8 g, Cholesterol: 28 mg, Sodium: 122 mg, Total Carbohydrate: 0.8 g, Dietary Fiber: 0.3 g, Total Sugars: 0.3 g, Protein: 10.7 g, Vitamin D: 0 mcg, Calcium: 16 mg, Iron: 1 mg, Potassium: 26 mg

Bacon Wrapped Asparagus

Servings: 2

Cooking Time: 30 Minutes

Ingredients:

1/3 cup heavy whipping cream

2 bacon slices, precooked

4 small spears asparagus

Salt, to taste

1 tablespoon butter

Directions:

Preheat the oven to 360 degrees F and grease a baking sheet with butter.

Meanwhile, mix cream, asparagus and salt in a bowl.

Wrap the asparagus in bacon slices and arrange them in the baking dish.

Transfer the baking dish in the oven and bake for about 20 minutes.

Remove from the oven and serve hot.

Place the bacon wrapped asparagus in a dish and set aside to cool for meal prepping. Divide it in 2 containers and cover the lid. Refrigerate for about 2 days and reheat in the microwave before serving.

Nutrition Info: Calories: 204 ;Carbohydrates: 1.4g;Protein: 5.9g;Fat: 19.3g;Sugar: 0.5g;Sodium: 291mg

Moroccan Spiced Stir-fried Beef With Butternut Squash And Chickpeas

Servings: 4
Cooking Time: 15 Minutes

Ingredients:

1 tablespoon olive oil, plus 2 teaspoons
1 pound precut butternut squash cut into ½-inch cubes
3 ounces scallions, white and green parts chopped (1 cup)
1 tablespoon water
¼ teaspoon baking soda
¾ pound flank steak, sliced across the grain into ⅛-inch thick slices
½ teaspoon garlic powder
¼ teaspoon ground ginger
¼ teaspoon turmeric
¼ teaspoon ground cumin
¼ teaspoon ground coriander
⅛ teaspoon cayenne pepper
⅛ teaspoon ground cinnamon
½ teaspoon kosher salt, divided

1 (14-ounce) can chickpeas, drained and rinsed

½ cup dried apricots, quartered

½ cup cilantro leaves, chopped

2 teaspoons freshly squeezed lemon juice

8 teaspoons sliced almonds

Directions:

Heat tablespoon of oil in a 12-inch skillet. Once the oil is hot, add the squash and scallions, and cook until the squash is tender, about 10 to 12 minutes.

Mix the water and baking soda together in a small prep bowl. Place the beef in a medium bowl, pour the baking-soda water over it, and mix to combine. Let it sit for 5 minutes.

In a small bowl, combine the garlic powder, ginger, turmeric, cumin, coriander, cayenne, cinnamon, and ¼ teaspoon of salt, then add the mixture to the beef. Stir to combine.

When the squash is tender, turn the heat off and add the remaining ¼ teaspoon of salt and the chickpeas, dried apricots, cilantro, and lemon juice to taste. Stir to combine. Place the contents of the pan in a bowl to cool.

Clean out the skillet and heat the remaining 2 teaspoons of oil over high heat. When the oil is hot, add the beef and cook until it is no longer pink, about 2 to 3 minutes.

Place 1¼ cups of the squash mixture and one quarter of the beef slices in each of 4 containers. Sprinkle 2 teaspoons of sliced almonds over each container.

STORAGE: Store covered containers in the refrigerator for up to 5 days.

Nutrition Info: Total calories: 404; Total fat: 14g; Saturated fat: 1g; Sodium: 355mg; Carbohydrates: 46g; Fiber: 12g; Protein: 27g

Herb-crusted Halibut

Servings: 4

Cooking Time: 25 Minutes

Ingredients:

Fresh parsley (.33 cup)

Fresh dill (.25 cup)

Fresh chives (.25 cup)

Lemon zest (1 tsp.)

Panko breadcrumbs (.75 cup)

Olive oil (1 tbsp.)

Freshly cracked black pepper (.25 tsp.)

Sea salt (1 tsp.)

Halibut fillets (4 - 6 oz.)

Directions:

Chop the fresh dill, chives, and parsley. Prepare a baking tray using a sheet of foil. Set the oven to reach 400° Fahrenheit.

Combine the salt, pepper, lemon zest, olive oil, chives, dill, parsley, and the breadcrumbs in a mixing bowl.

Rinse the halibut thoroughly. Use paper towels to dry it before baking.

Arrange the fish on the baking sheet. Spoon the crumbs over the fish and press it into each of the fillets.

Bake it until the top is browned and easily flaked or about 10 to 1minutes.

Nutrition Info: Calories: 273;Protein: 38 grams; Fat: 7 grams

Syrian Spiced Lentil, Barley, And Vegetable Soup

Servings: 5

Cooking Time: 40 Minutes

Ingredients:

1 tablespoon olive oil

1 small onion, chopped (about 2 cups)

2 medium carrots, peeled and chopped (about 1 cup)

1 celery stalk, chopped (about ½ cup)

1 teaspoon chopped garlic

1 teaspoon ground cumin

1 teaspoon ground coriander

1 teaspoon turmeric

⅛ teaspoon ground cinnamon

2 tablespoons tomato paste

¾ cup green lentils

¾ cup pearled barley

8 cups water

¾ teaspoon kosher salt

1 (5-ounce) package baby spinach leaves

2 teaspoons red wine vinegar

Directions:

Heat the oil in a soup pot on medium-high heat. When the oil is shimmering, add the onion, carrots, celery, and garlic and sauté for 8 minutes. Add the cumin, coriander, turmeric, cinnamon, and tomato paste and cook for 2 more minutes, stirring frequently.

Add the lentils, barley, water, and salt to the pot and bring to a boil. Turn the heat to low and simmer for minutes. Add the spinach and continue to simmer for 5 more minutes.

Add the vinegar and adjust the seasoning if needed. Spoon 2 cups of soup into each of 5 containers.

STORAGE: Store covered containers in the refrigerator for up to days.

Nutrition Info: Total calories: 273; Total fat: 4g; Saturated fat: 1g; Sodium: 459mg; Carbohydrates: 50g; Fiber: 1; Protein: 12g

Spinach Chicken

Servings: 2

Cooking Time: 20 Minutes

Ingredients:

2 garlic cloves, minced

2 tablespoons unsalted butter, divided

¼ cup parmesan cheese, shredded

¾ pound chicken tenders

¼ cup heavy cream

10 ounce frozen spinach, chopped

Salt and black pepper, to taste

Directions:

Heat tablespoon of butter in a large skillet and add chicken, salt and black pepper.

Cook for about 3 minutes on both sides and remove the chicken in a bowl.

Melt remaining butter in the skillet and add garlic, cheese, heavy cream and spinach.

Cook for about 2 minutes and transfer the chicken in it.

Cook for about minutes on low heat and dish out to immediately serve.

Place chicken in a dish and set aside to cool for meal prepping. Divide it in 2 containers and cover them. Refrigerate for about 3 days and reheat in microwave before serving.

Nutrition Info: Calories: 288 ;Carbohydrates: 3.6g;Protein: 27g;Fat: 18.3g;Sugar: 0.3g;Sodium: 192mg

Niçoise-style Tuna Salad With Olives & White Beans

Servings: 4

Cooking Time: 20-30 Minutes

Ingredients:

Green beans (.75 lb.)

Solid white albacore tuna (12 oz. can)

Great Northern beans (16 oz. can)

Sliced black olives (2.25 oz.)

Thinly sliced medium red onion (¼ of 1)

Hard-cooked eggs (4 large)

Dried oregano (1 tsp.)

Olive oil (6 tbsp.)

Black pepper and salt (as desired)

Finely grated lemon zest (.5 tsp.)

Water (.33 cup)

Lemon juice (3 tbsp.)

Directions:

Drain the can of tuna, Great Northern beans, and black olives. Trim and snap the green beans into halves.

Thinly slice the red onion. Cook and peel the eggs until hard-boiled.

Pour the water and salt into a skillet and add the beans. Place a top on the pot and switch the temperature setting to high. Wait for it to boil.

Once the beans are cooking, set a timer for five minutes. Immediately, drain and add the beans to a cookie sheet with a raised edge on paper towels to cool. Combine the onion, olives, white beans, and drained tuna. Mix them with the zest, lemon juice, oil, and oregano.

Dump the mixture over the salad and gently toss. Adjust the seasonings to your liking. Portion the tuna-bean salad with the green beans and eggs to serve.

Nutrition Info: Calories: 548;Protein: 36.3 grams;Fat: 30.3 grams

Whole-wheat Pasta With Roasted Red Pepper Sauce And Fresh Mozzarella

Servings: 4

Cooking Time: 40 Minutes

Ingredients:

3 large red bell peppers, seeds removed and cut in half

1 (10-ounce) container cherry tomatoes

2 teaspoons olive oil, plus 2 tablespoons

8 ounces whole-wheat penne or rotini

1 tablespoon plus 1 teaspoon apple cider vinegar

1 teaspoon chopped garlic

1½ teaspoons smoked paprika

¼ teaspoon kosher salt

½ cup packed fresh basil leaves, chopped

1 (8-ounce) container fresh whole-milk mozzarella balls (ciliegine), quartered

Directions:

Preheat the oven to 400°F and line a sheet pan with a silicone baking mat or parchment paper.

Place the peppers and tomatoes on the pan and toss with teaspoons of oil. Roast for 40 minutes.

While the peppers and tomatoes are roasting, cook the pasta according to the instructions on the box. Drain and place the pasta in a large mixing bowl.

When the peppers are cool enough to handle, peel the skin and discard. It's okay if you can't remove all the skin. Place the roasted peppers, vinegar, garlic, paprika, and salt and the remaining 2 tablespoons of oil in a blender and blend until smooth.

Add the pepper sauce, whole roasted tomatoes, basil, and mozzarella to the pasta and stir to combine.

Place a heaping 2 cups of pasta and sauce in each of 4 containers.

STORAGE: Store covered containers in the refrigerator for up to 5 days.

Nutrition Info: Total calories: 463; Total fat: 20g; Saturated fat: 7g; Sodium: 260mg; Carbohydrates: 54g; Fiber: 9g; Protein: 1

Greek Turkey Meatball Gyro With Tzatziki

Servings: 4
Cooking Time: 16 Minutes

Ingredients:
Turkey Meatball:
1 lb. ground turkey
1/4 cup finely diced red onion
2 garlic cloves, minced
1 tsp oregano
1 cup chopped fresh spinach
Salt, to taste
Pepper, to taste
2 tbsp olive oil
Tzatziki Sauce:
1/2 cup plain Greek yogurt
1/4 cup grated cucumber
2 tbsp lemon juice
1/2 tsp dry dill
1/2 tsp garlic powder
Salt, to taste

1/2 cup thinly sliced red onion

1 cup diced tomato

1 cup diced cucumber

4 whole wheat flatbreads

Directions:

In a large bowl, add in ground turkey, diced red onion, oregano, fresh spinach minced garlic, salt, and pepper

Using your hands mix all the ingredients together until the meat forms a ball and sticks together

Then using your hands, form meat mixture into 1" balls, making about 12 meatballs

In a large skillet over medium high heat, add the olive oil and then add the meatballs, cook each side for 3-minutes until they are browned on all sides, remove from the pan and allow it to rest

Allow the dish to cool completely

Distribute in the container, store for 2-3 days

To Serve: Reheat in the microwave for 1-2 minutes or until heated through. In the meantime, in a small bowl, combine the Greek yogurt, grated cucumber, lemon juice, dill, garlic powder, and salt to taste Assemble the gyros by taking the toasted flatbread, add 3 meatballs, sliced red onion, tomato, and cucumber. Top with Tzatziki sauce and serve!

Nutrition Info: Calories:429;Carbs: 3;Total Fat: 19g;Protein: 28g

Grilled Mediterranean Chicken Kebabs

Servings: 10
Cooking Time: 10 Minutes

Ingredients:

Chicken Kebabs:

3 chicken fillets, cut in 1-inch cubes

2 red bell peppers

2 green bell peppers

1 red onion

Chicken Kebab Marinade:

2/3 cup extra virgin olive oil, divided

Juice of 1 lemon, divided

6 clove of garlic, chopped, divided

4 tsp salt, divided

2 tsp freshly ground black pepper, divided

2 tsp paprika, divided

2 tsp thyme, divided

4 tsp oregano, divided

Directions:

In a bowl, mix 2 of all ingredients for the marinade- olive oils, lemon juice, garlic, salt, pepper, paprika, thyme and oregano in small bowl

Place the chicken in a ziplock bag and pour marinade over it, marinade in the fridge for about 30 minutes

In a separate ziplock bag, mix the other half of the marinade ingredients - olive oils, lemon juice, garlic, salt, pepper, paprika, thyme and oregano - add the vegetables and marinade for at least minutes

If you are using wood skewers, soak the skewers in water for about 20-30 minutes

Once done, thread the chicken and peppers and onions on the skewers in a pattern about 6 pieces of chicken with peppers and onion in between

Over an outdoor grill or indoor grill pan over medium-high heat, spray the grates lightly with oil

Grill the chicken for about 5 minutes on each side, or until cooked through, then allow to cool completely

Distribute among the containers, store for 2-3 days

To Serve: Reheat in the microwave for 1-2 minutes or until heated through, or cover in foil and reheat in the oven at 375 degrees F for 5 minutes

Recipe Notes: You can also bake the Mediterranean chicken skewers in the oven. Just preheat the oven to 425 F and place the chicken skewers on roasting racks that are over two foil-lined baking sheets. Bake for 15 minutes, turn over and bake for an additional 10 - 15 minutes on the other side, or until cooked through

Nutrition Info: Calories:228;Carbs: 5g;Total Fat: 17g;Protein: 14g

Kidney Beans Cilantro Salad

Servings: 6

Cooking Time: 30 Minutes

Ingredients:

1 15-ounce can kidney beans, rinsed and drained

½ English cucumber, chopped

1 medium heirloom tomato, chopped

1 bunch fresh cilantro, stems removed and chopped (about 1¼ cups)

1 red onion, chopped

lime juice, 1 large lime

3 tablespoons Dijon mustard

½ teaspoon fresh garlic paste

1 teaspoon sumac

salt

pepper

Directions:

Place kidney beans, vegetables, and cilantro in a serving bowl.

Cover, refrigerate and allow it to chill.

Before serving, in a small bowl, make the vinaigrette by adding limejuice, oil, fresh garlic, pepper, mustard, and sumac.

Pour the vinaigrette over the salad and give it a gentle stir.

Add some salt and pepper.

Serve!

Nutrition Info: Calories: 269, Total Fat: 1.3 g, Saturated Fat: 0.2 g, Cholesterol: 0 mg, Sodium: 112 mg, Total Carbohydrate: 49.3 g, Dietary Fiber: 12.g, Total Sugars: 3.9 g, Protein: 17.6 g, Vitamin D: 0 mcg, Calcium: 94 mg, Iron: 6 mg, Potassium: 1258 mg

Barley And Mushroom Soup

Servings: 6

Cooking Time: 30 Minutes

Ingredients:

2 tablespoons of olive oil

1 cup chopped carrots

6 cups vegetable broth, no salt added, and low sodium is best

¼ cup red wine

5 tablespoons parmesan cheese, grated

½ teaspoon thyme

1 cup chopped onion

5 cups chopped mushrooms

1 cup pearled barley, uncooked

2 tablespoons tomato paste

Directions:

Place a stockpot on your stove and turn the temperature of the range to medium heat.

Pour in the oil and let it warm up and start to simmer.

Combine the carrots and onion. Let them cook for 5 to 8 minutes while frequently stirring the ingredients together.

Add the mushroom and turn the heat up to medium-high. Stir and cook for a few minutes.

Pour in the broth and stir the ingredients for a few seconds.

Add in the wine, barley, thyme, and tomato paste. Stir everything together and then set the cover on the pot.

When the soup starts to boil, stir and reduce the heat to medium-low.

Cover the soup again and set your timer for 15 minutes, but don't leave it alone. You will want to stir a few times, so all ingredients become well incorporated.

Once the dish becomes fragrant and the barley is completely cooked, turn off the heat and serve in bowls. Sprinkle the cheese on top for added taste and enjoy!

Nutrition Info: calories: 236, fats: 7 grams, carbohydrates: 35 grams, protein: 8 grams.

Pan-seared Scallops With Pepper & Onions In Anchovy Oil

Servings: 4
Cooking Time: 45 Minutes

Ingredients:

Olive oil (.33 cup)
Anchovy fillets (2 oz. can)
Jumbo sea scallops (1 lb.)
Orange & red bell pepper (1 large of each)
Red onion (1)
Garlic (2 cloves)
Lime zest (1 tsp.)
Lemon zest (1.5 tsp.)
Kosher salt & pepper (1 pinch of each)
Garnish: Fresh parsley (8 sprigs)

Directions:

Coarsely chop the peppers and onions. Mince the garlic and anchovy fillet. Zest/mince the lime and lemon.
Heat the oil and anchovies in a large skillet using a med-high temperature setting.

After the anchovies are sizzling, toss in the scallops, and simmer them for about two minutes - without stirring.

Toss the bell peppers, garlic, red onion, lime zest, lemon zest, salt, and pepper into a mixing container. Sprinkle the mixture over the scallops. Cook until they have browned (2 min..)

Flip the scallops, stir, and continue cooking until the scallops have browned thoroughly (4-min..)

Top it off using sprigs of parsley before serving.

Nutrition Info: Calories: 368;Protein: 24.2 grams; Fat: 23.9 grams

Spinach Salad With Blood Orange Vinaigrette

Servings: 6
Cooking Time: 10 Minutes

Ingredients:

½ cup fresh blood orange juice

1/3 cup extra-virgin olive oil

2 tablespoons sherry reserve vinegar

1 tablespoon fresh grated ginger

1 teaspoon garlic powder

1 teaspoon ground sumac

salt

pepper

1/3 cup dried apricots, chopped

2 tablespoons sherry reserve vinegar

2 loaves pita bread

2/3 cup vegetable oil

1/3 cup raw unsalted almonds

1/3 cup raw sliced almonds

½ teaspoon sumac

½ teaspoon paprika

salt

4 cups baby spinach

3 cups frisee lettuce, chopped

2 shallots, thinly sliced

1-2 blood oranges, peeled and sliced crosswise

Directions:

In a small bowl, soak the dried apricots in the sherry-reserved vinegar for about 5 minutes.

Drain apricots and set aside.

Toast pita bread until crispy and break into pieces.

Heat vegetable oil in a frying pan over medium-high heat.

Add broken pitas and almonds and fry them for a while.

Add sliced up almonds, sumac, and paprika, and toss everything well.

Remove from heat once the almonds show a golden brown color.

Place on paper towels and allow to drain.

In a mixing bowl, add baby spinach, shallots, apricots, frisee lettuce.

Prepare the vinaigrette by taking a bowl and whisking in all blood orange vinaigrette Ingredients: listed above.

Before serving, dress the salad with the prepared orange vinaigrette and toss well.

Add fried pita chips and almonds and toss again.

Serve into individual bowls with a garnish of two blood orange slices.

Enjoy!

Nutrition Info: Calories: 462, Total Fat: 41.2 g, Saturated Fat: 6.9 g, Cholesterol: 0 mg, Sodium: 110 mg, Total Carbohydrate: 22.6 g, Dietary Fiber: 6.8 g, Total Sugars: 6.8 g, Protein: 6.1 g, Vitamin D: 0 mcg, Calcium: 163 mg, Iron: 3 mg, Potassium: 702 mg

Lasagna Tortellini Soup

Servings: 6

Cooking Time: 6 Hours

Ingredients:

1 lb extra lean ground beef

1 package (16 oz) frozen cheese filled tortellini

3 cups beef broth

1/2 cup yellow onion, chopped

2 cloves garlic, minced

1 can (28 oz) crushed tomatoes

1 can (14.5 oz) petite diced tomatoes

1 can (6 oz) tomato paste

1 can (10.75 oz) tomato condensed soup

1 tsp white sugar

1 ½ tsp dried basil

1 tsp Italian seasoning

1/2 tbsp salt, to taste

1/4 tsp pepper

Optional:

4 tbsp fresh parsley

1/2 tsp fennel seeds

Toppings:

Freshly grated Parmesan cheese

Large spoonful of ricotta cheese

Directions:

In a large skillet over medium heat, brown the ground beef until cooked through

Add the onion and garlic in the last few minutes of the cooking

While the beef is cooking, pour in the crushed tomatoes, petite diced tomatoes, tomato paste, and tomato condensed soup in the slow cooker. - Don't drain the cans!

Add in the sugar, the dried basil, fennel, Italian seasoning, salt, and pepper, adjust to taste

Stir in the cooked ground beef with onions and garlic

Add in the beef broth – or dissolved beef bouillon cubes into boiling water

Cook on high for 3-4 hours or low for 5-hours.

15-20 minutes before you are ready to serve the soup, add in the frozen tortellini

Set the slow cooker to high and allow the tortellini to heat through

Allow to cool, then distribute the soup into the container and store in the fridge for up to 3 days

To Serve: Reheat in the microwave or on the stove top, top with freshly grated Parmesan cheese, a large spoonful of ricotta cheese, extra seasonings and freshly chopped parsley.

Nutrition Info: Calories:499;Total Fat: 17g;Total Carbs: 53g;Fiber: 8g;Protein: 34g

Greek Quinoa Bowls

Servings: 2

Cooking Time: 12 Minutes

Ingredients:

1 cup quinoa

1 ½ cups water

1 cup chopped green bell pepper

1 cup chopped red bell pepper

1/3 cup crumbled feta cheese

1/4 cup extra virgin olive oil

2-3 tbsp apple cider vinegar

Salt, to taste

Pepper, to taste

1-2 tbsp fresh parsley

To Serve:

Hummus

Pita wedges

Olives

Fresh tomatoes

Sliced or chopped avocado

Lemon wedges

Directions:

Rinse and drain the quinoa using a mesh strainer or sieve. Place a medium saucepan to medium heat and lightly toast the quinoa to remove any excess water. Stir as it toasts for just a few minutes, to add a nuttiness and fluff to the quinoa

Then add the water, set burner to high, and bring to a boil.

Once boiling, reduce heat to low and simmer, covered with the lid slightly ajar, for 12-1minutes or until quinoa is fluffy and the liquid have been absorbed

In the meantime, mix whisk together olive oil, apple cider vinegar, salt, and pepper to make the dressing, store in the fridge until ready to serve

Add in the red bell peppers, green bell peppers, and parsley

Give the quinoa a little fluff with a fork, remove from the pot

Allow to cool completely

Distribute among the containers, store for 2-3 days

To Serve: Reheat in the microwave for 1-2 minutes or until heated through.

Pour the dressing over the quinoa bowl, toss add the feta cheese. Season with additional salt and pepper to taste, if desired. Enjoy!

Nutrition Info: Calories:645;Carbs: 61g;Total Fat: 37g;Protein: 16g

Salmon Stew

Servings: 2

Cooking Time: 20 Minutes

Ingredients:

1 pound salmon fillet, sliced

1 onion, chopped

Salt, to taste

1 tablespoon butter, melted

1 cup fish broth

½ teaspoon red chili powder

Directions:

Season the salmon fillets with salt and red chili powder.

Put butter and onions in a skillet and sauté for about 3 minutes.

Add seasoned salmon and cook for about 2 minutes on each side.

Add fish broth and secure the lid.

Cook for about 7 minutes on medium heat and open the lid.

Dish out and serve immediately.

Transfer the stew in a bowl and keep aside to cool for meal prepping. Divide the mixture into 2 containers. Cover the containers and refrigerate for about 2 days. Reheat in the microwave before serving.

Nutrition Info: Calories: 272 ;Carbohydrates: 4.4g;Protein: 32.1g;Fat: 14.2g ;Sugar: 1.9g;Sodium: 275mg

Balsamic Chicken And Veggie Skewers

Servings: 4
Cooking Time: 25 Minutes

Ingredients:

1 pound boneless, skinless chicken breasts, cut into 1-inch cubes

⅓ cup balsamic vinegar

4 tablespoons olive oil, divided

4 teaspoons dried Italian herbs, divided

2 teaspoons garlic powder, divided

2 teaspoons onion powder, divided

8 ounces whole button or cremini mushrooms, stems removed

1 large red bell pepper, cut into 1-inch squares

1 small red onion, quartered and layers pulled apart

1 large zucchini, sliced into ½-inch rounds

¾ teaspoon kosher salt

8 (11¾-inch) wooden or metal skewers, soaked in water for at least 1 hour if wooden

Directions:

Preheat the oven to 450°F. Line a sheet pan with aluminum foil.

Place the chicken in a gallon-size resealable bag along with the balsamic vinegar, tablespoons of oil, 2 teaspoons of Italian herbs, 1 teaspoon of garlic powder, and 1 teaspoon of onion powder. Seal the bag and make sure all the pieces of chicken are coated with marinade.

In a second resealable bag, place the mushrooms, bell pepper, onion, and zucchini and the remaining 2 tablespoons of oil, 2 teaspoons of Italian herbs, 1 teaspoon of garlic powder, and 1 teaspoon of onion powder. Seal the bag and shake to make sure the veggies are coated.

Refrigerate both bags and marinate for at least 2 hours. Thread the chicken and veggies on 8 skewers, alternating both chicken and veggies on each skewer. Place 6 skewers vertically in the center of the pan, 1 horizontally at the top, and 1 at the bottom. Sprinkle half the salt over the skewers, then flip over and sprinkle the skewers with the remaining salt.

Bake for 15 minutes, carefully flip the skewers, then bake for another 10 minutes. Cool.

If you have containers long enough to fit the skewers, place 2 skewers directly in each of 4 containers. If not, break the skewers in half or slide the meat and veggies off the skewers.

STORAGE: Store covered containers in the refrigerator for up to 5 days.

Nutrition Info: Total calories: 224; Total fat: 10g; Saturated fat: 2g; Sodium: 631mg; Carbohydrates: 11g; Fiber: 3g; Protein: 27g

Pesto Chicken And Tomato Zoodles

Servings: 4

Cooking Time: 15 Minutes

Ingredients:

3 Zucchini, inspiralized

2 boneless skinless chicken breasts

1 1/2 cup cherry tomatoes

2 tsp olive oil

1/2 tsp salt

Store brought Pesto or Homemade Basil Pesto

Salt, to taste

Pepper, to taste

Directions:

Preheat grill to medium high heat

Season both sides of the chicken with salt and pepper

Place cherry tomatoes in a small bowl, add the olive oil and 1/2 tsp salt, and toss the tomatoes

In the meantime, inspiralize the zucchini, set aside

Pour the pesto over the zucchini noodles, using salad toss or tongs, mix the pesto in with the zoodles until it is completely combined

Place the chicken on the grill and grill each side for 5-7 minutes, or until cooked through

Place cherry tomatoes in a grill basket and grill for 5 minutes, until tomatoes burst

Remove the tomatoes and chicken from the grill, slice the chicken and place both sliced chicken and tomatoes into the pesto zoodles bowl

allow the dish to cool completely

Distribute among the containers, store for 2-3 days

To Serve: Reheat in the microwave for 1-2 minutes or until heated through. Enjoy

Nutrition Info: Calories:396;Carbs: 8g;Total Fat: 30g;Protein: 18g

Broiled Herb Sole With Cauliflower Mashed Potatoes

Servings: 4

Cooking Time: 16 Minutes

Ingredients:

12 ounces cauliflower florets, cut into 1-inch pieces

1 (12-ounce) Yukon Gold potato, cut into ¾-inch pieces (do not peel)

2 tablespoons olive oil

¼ teaspoon kosher salt

2 teaspoons olive oil, plus more to grease the pan

3 tablespoons chopped parsley

3 tablespoons chopped fresh dill

1 tablespoon freshly squeezed lemon juice

½ teaspoon chopped garlic

1¼ pounds boneless, skinless sole or tilapia

¼ teaspoon kosher salt

4 lemon wedges, for serving

Directions:

TO MAKE THE CAULIFLOWER MASHED POTATOES

Pour enough water into a saucepan that it reaches ½ inch up the side of the pan. Turn the heat to high and bring the water to a boil. Add the cauliflower and potatoes, and cover the pan. Steam for 10 minutes or until the veggies are very tender.

Drain the vegetables if water remains in the pan. Transfer the veggies to a large bowl and add the olive oil and salt. Taste and add an additional pinch of salt if you need it.

Once the veggies have cooled, scoop ¾ cup of cauliflower mashed potatoes into each of containers.

TO MAKE THE SOLE

Preheat the oven to the high broiler setting. Line a sheet pan with foil and lightly grease the pan with oil or cooking spray.

Mix the oil, parsley, dill, lemon juice, and garlic in a small bowl. Pat the fish with paper towels to remove excess moisture and place on the lined sheet pan. Sprinkle the salt over the fish, then spread the herb mixture over the fish. Broil for about 6 minutes or until the fish is flaky. If your fish is very thin, broil for 5 minutes.

When everything has cooled, place one quarter of the fish in each of the 4 cauliflower containers. Serve with lemon wedges.

STORAGE: Store covered containers in the refrigerator for up to 4 days.

Nutrition Info: Total calories: 291; Total fat: 11g; Saturated fat: 1g; Sodium: 423mg; Carbohydrates: 20g; Fiber: 2g; Protein: 29g

Citrus Poached Lovely Salmon

Servings: 4

Cooking Time: 40 Minutes

Ingredients:

6 cups water

½ cup freshly squeezed lemon juice

Juice of 1 lime

Zest of 1 lime

1 sweet onion, thinly sliced

1 cup celery leaves, coarsely chopped

1 tablespoon fresh dill, chopped

1 tablespoon fresh thyme, chopped

2 dried bay leaves

½ teaspoon black peppercorns

½ teaspoon sea salt

1 (24 ounce salmon side, skinned and deboned, cut into 4 pieces

Directions:

Take a large saucepan and place it over medium-high heat

Stir water, lemon, lime juice, lem0on juice, lime zest, onion, celery, greens, thyme, dill and bay leaves

Strain the liquid through fine mesh sieve, discard any solids

Pour strained poaching liquid into large skillet over low heat

Bring to a simmer

Add fish and cover skillet, poach for 10 minutes until opaque

Remove salmon from liquid and serve

Enjoy!

Meal Prep/Storage Options: Store in airtight containers in your fridge for 1-3 days.

Nutrition Info: Calories: 248;Fat: 11g;Carbohydrates: 4g;Protein: 34g

GREAT MEDITERRANEAN DIET RECIPES

Herb rice

Preparation time: 5 minutes

Cooking time: 20 minutes

Servings: 4

Ingredients:

1 tsp salt

2 Tbsp butter

1 tsp onion black pepper juice

3 cup chicken broth

1 tsp garlic

1/4 cup lemon juice

1.5 cup basmati rice

1/2 tsp rosemary, basil, dill, parsley, oregano, thyme

Directions :

Melt butter on moderate heat & add salt & black pepper powder. Keep stirring till the onion is softened.

Now add garlic & cook (1 min)

Add chicken broth & lemon juice with herb along with rice.

Keep stirring until mixed.

Now, wait for a boil, cover & lower heat.

Keep cooking until rice is well softened & garnish with herbs if required.

Serve & enjoy.

Nutrition Info: Calories: 227 kcal Fat: 0 g Protein: 4 g Carbs: 49 g Fiber: 3 g

Pecorino pasta with sausage and tomato

Preparation time: 20 minutes
Cooking time: 20 minutes
Servings: 4

Ingredients:

2 tsp olive oil

1 cup sliced onion

8 oz penne

8 oz Italian sausage

6 tbsp grated Romano cheese

1/4 tsp salt

2 tsp garlic

1 1/4 lb tomatoes

1/8 tsp black pepper

1/4 cup torn basil leaves

Directions :

Boil & drain pasta. Keep the boiled pasta aside. Now at a full flame, heat a skillet, which should be nonstick. Take oil in a pan & add sausage and onion to it. Cook for about two minutes. Now remove from stove & add pasta, salt, black pepper powder & cheese. Add oil to a pan, swirl to coat.

Sprinkle remaining 1/4th cup of cheese and serve

Nutrition Info: Calories: 389 kcal Fat: 10 g Protein: 21.6 g Carbs: 53.5 g Fiber: 4.5 g

Pesto pasta and shrimp

Preparation time: 10 minutes

Cooking time: 10 minutes

Servings: 3

Ingredients:

10 oz spaghetti

3/4 cup basil pesto

1 lb shrimp

1 tbsp olive oil

1 tsp Italian seasoning

Salt to taste

Black pepper to taste

1/4 cup parmesan cheese

Directions :

Bring a pot of salted water to a boil and cook the pasta. While the pasta is cooking, prepare the shrimp. Heat the olive oil in a pan over high heat.

Add the shrimp and sprinkle with Italian seasoning, salt, and pepper.

Cook for 2-4 minutes or until shrimp is just pink and opaque. Turn off the heat.

Drain the pasta and add it to the pan with the shrimp. Stir in the pesto.

Add the cherry tomatoes and parmesan cheese to the pan.

Garnish with parsley if desired.

Nutrition Info: Calories: 627 kcal Fat: 30 g Protein: 40 g Carbs: 57 g Fiber: 5 g

Feta tomato sea bass

Preparation time: 10 minutes

Cooking time: 10 minutes

Servings: 4

Ingredients:

2 oz dry white wine

2 tbsp lemon juice

32 oz sea bass fillets

4 oz feta cheese

Five ripe tomatoes

5 tbsp olive oil

2 tbsp butter

2 tbsp basil

Three garlic cloves

1 tbsp oregano

Salt & pepper

Directions :

Take fish & rub salt & pepper over it. Heat the pan & add olive oil.

Put the fish in a pan. Cook it until it is golden brown. Add basil, cheese, lemon juice, tomatoes & garlic. Bake 12-15 minutes at 400 deg. Take the dish out and finish it with butter. The dish is ready. Now serve and enjoy.

Nutrition Info: Calories: 549 kcal Fat: 34 g Protein: 48.1 g Carbs: 9.9 g Fiber: 2.3 g

Bulgur Vegetable Salad

Preparation time: 15 minutes

Cooking time: 0 minute

Servings: 5

Ingredients:

1 cup Cooked Bulgur

1 cup broccoli Chopped

1 cup cauliflower Chopped

One chopped red bell pepper

1 Scallion Chopped

2 tbsp chopped basil leaves

lemon juice & zest

1 tbsp olive oil

Black pepper according to taste

Directions : In a large bowl, mix the broccoli, bulgur, bell pepper, scallion, cauliflower, basil, lemon juice, olive oil, & lemon zest. Flavor with pepper. Toss again & serve.

Nutrition Info: Calories: 106 kcal Fat: 3 g Protein: 3 g Carbs: 18 g Fiber: 4 g

Cauliflower Breadsticks

Preparation Time: 7 minutes

Cook Time: 30 minutes

Serving: 12

Ingredients

4 lb cauliflower

Two egg whites

1.5 cup Mozzarella cheese shredded

Italian seasoning 1 tsp

Pinch of salt

1/4 tsp black pepper

Marinara sauce for dipping

Cooking spray

Directions : Toast blended cauliflower in oven at 375 degrees for 20 minutes. Mix roasted cauliflower with egg whites, cheese, herbs, salt, pepper in a bowl. Bake the mixture in the oven at 450 degrees for 18 minutes. Bring in sticks, shape, and serve.

Nutrition Info: Calories: 51 kcal Fat: 0.2 g Protein: 4.6 g Carbs: 5 g Fiber: 1 g

Cheesecake Ice Cream

Preparation Time: 20 Minutes

Cooking Time: 20 Minutes

Serving: 1.5 quarts

Ingredients

1 cup milk

Two eggs

2.5 cups cream

1 tsp vanilla extract

1-1/4 cups sugar

12 oz. cream cheese

1 tbsp lemon juice

Directions : Melt sugar in cream and milk mixture. Whisk in egg and transfer in a pan. Cook over medium flame. Remove from flame and mix in cream cheese. Cool the mixture and stir in lemon juice and vanilla extract. Refrigerate it for 120 minutes and serve.

Nutrition Info: Calories: 272 kcal Fat: 16 g Protein: 6 g Carbs: 24 g Fiber: 0 g

Vanilla Custard

Preparation Time: 10 minutes

Cooking Time: 20 minutes

Serving: 4

Ingredients

1 tbsp corn-flour

1/3 cup sugar

1 Vanilla Bean

1 cup milk

Four yolks of egg

1 cup cream

Directions : Cook vanilla, milk, and cream in a saucepan with continuous stirring. Pour cream mixture over egg, sugar, and corn flour mixture in a bowl. Cook until the required thickness is achieved.
Cook and serve.

Nutrition Info: Calories: 272 kcal Fat: 16 g Protein: 6 g Carbs: 24 g Fiber: 0 g

Chocolate Fruit Kebabs

Servings: 6

Cooking Time: 30 Minutes

Ingredients:

24 blueberries

12 strawberries with the green leafy top part removed

12 green or red grapes, seedless

12 pitted cherries

8 ounces chocolate

Directions:

Line a baking sheet with a piece of parchment paper and place 6, - inch long wooden skewers on top of the paper.

Start by threading a piece of fruit onto the skewers. You can create and follow any pattern that you like with the ingredients. An example pattern is 1 strawberry, 1 cherry, blueberries, 2 grapes. Repeat the pattern until all of the fruit is on the skewers.

In a saucepan on medium heat, melt the chocolate. Stir continuously until the chocolate has melted completely.

Carefully scoop the chocolate into a plastic sandwich bag and twist the bag closed starting right above the chocolate.

Snip the corner of the bag with scissors.

Drizzle the chocolate onto the kebabs by squeezing it out of the bag.

Put the baking pan into the freezer for 20 minutes.

Serve and enjoy!

Nutrition Info: calories: 254, fats: 15 grams, carbohydrates: 28 grams, protein: 4 grams.

SAUCES AND DRESSINGS RECIPES

Chunky Roasted Cherry Tomato And Basil Sauce

Servings: 1⅓ Cups
Cooking Time: 40 Minutes

Ingredients:

2 pints cherry tomatoes (20 ounces total)

2 teaspoons olive oil, plus 3 tablespoons

¼ teaspoon kosher salt

½ teaspoon chopped garlic

¼ cup fresh basil leaves

Directions:

Preheat the oven to 350°F. Line a sheet pan with a silicone baking mat or parchment paper.

Place the tomatoes on the lined sheet pan and toss with teaspoons of oil. Roast for 40 minutes, shaking the pan halfway through.

While the tomatoes are still warm, place them in a medium mixing bowl and add the salt, the garlic, and the remaining tablespoons of oil. Mash the tomatoes with the back of a fork. Stir in the fresh basil.

Scoop the sauce into a container and refrigerate.

STORAGE: Store the covered container in the refrigerator for up to days.

Nutrition Info: Per Serving (⅓ cup): Total calories: 141; Total fat: 13g; Saturated fat: 2g; Sodium: 158mg; Carbohydrates: 7g; Fiber: 2g; Protein: 1g

Basil, Almond, And Celery Heart Pesto

Servings: 1 Cup
Cooking Time: 10 Minutes

Ingredients:

½ cup raw, unsalted almonds
3 cups fresh basil leaves, (about 1½ ounces)
½ cup chopped celery hearts with leaves
¼ teaspoon kosher salt
1 tablespoon freshly squeezed lemon juice
¼ cup olive oil
3 tablespoons water

Directions:

Place the almonds in the bowl of a food processor and process until they look like coarse sand.

Add the basil, celery hearts, salt, lemon juice, oil and water and process until smooth. The sauce will be somewhat thick. If you would like a thinner sauce, add more water, oil, or lemon juice, depending on your taste preference.

Scoop the pesto into a container and refrigerate.

STORAGE: Store the covered container in the refrigerator for up to 2 weeks. Pesto may be frozen for up to 6 months.

Nutrition Info: Per Serving (¼ cup): Total calories: 231; Total fat: 22g; Saturated fat: 3g; Sodium: 178mg; Carbohydrates: 6g; Fiber: 3g; Protein: 4g

Sweet And Spicy Green Pumpkin Seeds

Servings: 2 Cups
Cooking Time: 15 Minutes

Ingredients:

2 cups raw green pumpkin seeds (pepitas)
1 egg white, beaten until frothy
3 tablespoons honey
1 tablespoon chili powder
¼ teaspoon cayenne pepper
1 teaspoon ground cinnamon
¼ teaspoon kosher salt

Directions:

Preheat the oven to 350°F. Line a sheet pan with a silicone baking mat or parchment paper.

In a medium bowl, mix all the ingredients until the seeds are well coated. Place on the lined sheet pan in a single, even layer.

Bake for 15 minutes. Cool the seeds on the sheet pan, then peel clusters from the baking mat and break apart into small pieces.

Place ¼ cup of seeds in each of 8 small containers or resealable sandwich bags.

STORAGE: Store covered containers or resealable bags at room temperature for up to days.

Nutrition Info: Per Serving (¼ cup): Total calories: 209; Total fat: 15g; Saturated fat: 3g; Sodium: 85mg; Carbohydrates: 11g; Fiber: 2g; Protein: 10g

Chermoula Sauce

Servings: 1 Cup
Cooking Time: 10 Minutes

Ingredients:
1 cup packed parsley leaves
1 cup cilantro leaves
½ cup mint leaves
1 teaspoon chopped garlic
½ teaspoon ground cumin
½ teaspoon ground coriander
½ teaspoon smoked paprika
⅛ teaspoon cayenne pepper
⅛ teaspoon kosher salt
3 tablespoons freshly squeezed lemon juice
3 tablespoons water
½ cup extra-virgin olive oil

Directions:
Place all the ingredients in a blender or food processor and blend until smooth.
Pour the chermoula into a container and refrigerate.

STORAGE: Store the covered container in the refrigerator for up to 5 days.

Nutrition Info: Per Serving (¼ cup): Total calories: 257; Total fat: 27g; Saturated fat: ; Sodium: 96mg; Carbohydrates: 4g; Fiber: 2g; Protein: 1g

Pesto Deviled Eggs With Sun-dried Tomatoes

Servings: 5
Cooking Time: 15 Minutes

Ingredients:

5 large eggs

3 tablespoons prepared pesto

¼ teaspoon white vinegar

2 tablespoons low-fat (2%) plain Greek yogurt

5 teaspoons sliced sun-dried tomatoes

Directions:

Place the eggs in a saucepan and cover with water. Bring the water to a boil. As soon as the water starts to boil, place a lid on the pan and turn the heat off. Set a timer for minutes.

When the timer goes off, drain the hot water and run cold water over the eggs to cool.

Peel the eggs, slice in half vertically, and scoop out the yolks. Place the yolks in a medium mixing bowl and add the pesto, vinegar, and yogurt. Mix well, until creamy.

Scoop about 1 tablespoon of the pesto-yolk mixture into each egg half. Top each with ½ teaspoon of sun-dried tomatoes.

Place 2 stuffed egg halves in each of separate containers.

STORAGE: Store covered containers in the refrigerator for up to 5 days.

Nutrition Info: Total calories: 124; Total fat: 9g; Saturated fat: 2g; Sodium: 204mg; Carbohydrates: 2g; Fiber: <1g; Protein: 8g

North African Spiced Sautéed Cabbage

Servings: 4

Cooking Time: 10 Minutes

Ingredients:

2 teaspoons olive oil

1 small head green cabbage (about 1½ to 2 pounds), cored and thinly sliced

1 teaspoon ground coriander

1 teaspoon garlic powder

½ teaspoon caraway seeds

½ teaspoon ground cumin

¼ teaspoon kosher salt

Pinch red chili flakes (optional—if you don't like heat, omit it)

1 teaspoon freshly squeezed lemon juice

Directions:

Heat the oil in a -inch skillet over medium-high heat. Once the oil is hot, add the cabbage and cook down for 3 minutes. Add the coriander, garlic powder, caraway seeds, cumin, salt, and chili flakes (if using) and stir to combine. Continue cooking the cabbage for about 7 more minutes.

Stir in the lemon juice and cool.

Place 1 heaping cup of cabbage in each of 4 containers.

STORAGE: Store covered containers in the refrigerator for up to 5 days.

Nutrition Info: Total calories: 69; Total fat: 3g; Saturated fat: <1g; Sodium: 178mg; Carbohydrates: 11g; Fiber: 4g; Protein: 3g

www.ingramcontent.com/pod-product-compliance
Ingram Content Group UK Ltd.
Pitfield, Milton Keynes, MK11 3LW, UK
UKHW020048130126
10059UKWH00060B/410